Breast Cancer in Men

Men Who Develop Breast Cancer

TABLE OF CONTENTS

Male breast cancer is a cancer of men's breast tissue. Breast cancer is often seen as a disease for women, but this happens to a large extent. Understanding the symptoms of cancer is critical. The illness in elderly men is more severe, but it can happen at any age.

Men who are diagnosed with cancer are well-placed to cure if detected early. Cancer symptoms should not be ignored. The most common symptom is a breast lump. Most cases are diagnosed when the condition is advanced.

Some of its signs are: a lump that is painless in nature, thickening of the breast tissue, dimpling, swelling, redness and scaling that takes place on the skin covering the breast.

The nipple might transform inside. It is also possible to rot and scale.

There may be discharge from the nipple. When signs and symptoms occur, see your doctor.

The causes of cancer are not very clear. Abnormally developing breast cells are a sign of cancer. These cells tend to split faster than healthy cells. The growing cells form a tumor that can spread to the surrounding tissue, lymph nodes, or other parts of the body.

Each person is born with a certain amount of breast tissue. The tissue consists of lobules, which produce milk. The lobules are gateways that carry milk to the nipples. In comparison to men, women develop much more breast tissue during puberty. Because of the low presence of breast tissue, men may develop breast cancer.

Breast cancer forms in men are as follows:

1. Ductal carcinoma is the most common form of breast cancer. Almost all cancers emerge from the breast canals.

2. Milk-producing gland cancer: Lobular carcinoma is not common among men, since it has few breast tissue lobules.

3. In some instances, breast cancer can originate in the ducts but spread to the nipples. This may cause the nipple skin to become scaly. This is also known as the illness of Paget.

Genes may increase the risk of breast cancer in some cases. People inherit their parents' genetic mutations that increase the risk of breast cancer. The risk of breast or prostate cancer may increase with a mutation in a particular gene known as BRCA2. This gene generally helps prevent cancer by generating proteins that stop cells from growing abnormally. Nevertheless, they switch their positions when they experience changes.

IDENTIFICATION OF MEN'S BREAST CANCER SYMPTOMS

Breast cancer Symptoms in men
There is a common misunderstanding that men are unable to grow breast cancer. Men often neglect or confuse signs of cancer for other diseases. Factors like social stigma and humiliation lead to the growing reluctance of men to detect breast cancer. The incidence of male (breast) cancer is close to that of women. Males aged 60 to 70 are more likely to develop this type of cancer than any other age group.

The latest estimate from the American Cancer Society for male breast cancer indicates that about 1,910 cases and around 440 deaths will be diagnosed in 2009. Around one percent of cases of cancer affect men as breast cancer. The risk of developing this type of cancer is approximately one in a thousand. Recent studies also show that the outlook for both men and women of this type of cancer remains the same, and the expectation is based on what point the cancer has been diagnosed.

As with any other cancer, early detection and treatment are essential to the survival of a patient. Men are therefore advised to be more aware of the signs and symptoms of cancer. Educating men to fight the social stigma created by cancer often helps men battle this type of cancer.

Diagnosis of breast cancer in men: Awareness of symptoms and signs of cancer are very helpful in providing people with this breast cancer with the earliest possible diagnosis and care available. Here are some signs of breast cancer.

Disturbing swelling or breast thickening, color and redness of nipple and surroundings, and indentation or retraction in the nipple area. The risk of breast cancer is compounded by factors that increase the risk of breast cancer. Some of which are uncontrollable, like genetics and age. Moreover, certain risk factors, such as poor diet, alcohol and smoking, can be tracked so that we know what we should avoid. Below is a list of risk factors for breast cancer in men.

The average age of diagnosis for male breast cancer is 67 years and in men between the ages of 60 and 70.

One in five men with breast cancer had a woman parent who also suffered from breast cancer.

Those who have received radiation on the chest are more likely to have breast cancer.

Around 5-10% of male breast cancers are hereditary. Genetic defects in the genes CHEK-2, p53, BRCA2 and BRCA1 increase a person's risk of cancer. Such genes usually help to prevent cancer by preventing abnormal cell growth.

Those that had a history of Klinefelter syndrome had an extra X chromosome that resulted in lower levels of male and female hormones.

Those who have taken estrogen-related drugs are more vulnerable to breast cancer. It is known that breast cancer cells have estrogen receptors that improve the ability of cancer to progress.

Liver diseases are also a risk when the body's estrogen increases and the activity of androgen decreases when a person is affected by liver diseases, such as liver cirrhosis.

Obesity is also likely because of the increased number of fat cells in male breast cancer. Fat cells contain androgen estrogen, thus increasing the body's estrogen concentration.

Excessive alcohol consumption also causes breast cancer in men, primarily because alcohol consumption increases liver disorders and the accumulation of fat.

Treatment options for breast cancer in men: Many treatment methods for men with breast cancer are available. Such approaches are not different from those for women. Cancer phase is used to assess a patient's best treatment choice for breast cancer. Here are some of the available treatment choices.

Surgery–Several options are used to remove breast cancer in men, such as simple mastectomy, modified radical mastectomy, and sentinel lymph node biopsy. Simple mastectomy entails the removal of the lobules, ducts, fatty tissue, and skin, including the nipple and arselet.

The surgeon removes the entire breast and part of the subarmed lymph nodes in a modified radical mastectomy. If the cancer has spread to this area, the surgeon may also remove chest wall muscle. The lymph nodes are checked to test for the spread of cancer and for additional treatment.

Sentinel lymph node biopsy is a technique designed to identify sentinel nodes, which are removed from a breast tumor. Sentinel nodes are removed to monitor the progression of cancer in other lymph nodes for biopsy. This technique decreases the risk of complications because it is necessary to remove a single node for review.

Radiation Therapy— High-energy X-rays are used during radiation therapy to kill cancer cells. A radiation oncologist usually performs treatment before surgery to shrink the tumor or after surgery to remove other cancer cells. Radiation therapy is often painless but may cause fatigue in people undergoing therapy and breast tenderness.

Chemotherapy Hormone Therapy: Biological Chemotherapy requires the use of medications to kill cancer cells that have spread to other parts of the body after a breast cancer procedure. Treatment is typically planned for three to six months every two or three weeks after the procedure.

Chemotherapy can be administered intravenously or in the form of a tablet. Many patients opt for oral chemotherapy because it eliminates the need to visit the hospital and is available at home.

Some chemotherapies aim to reduce damage to healthy cells by cancer. Nonetheless, side effects such as hair loss, nausea, vomiting and cognitive impairment can occur.

Estrogen receptor positive breast cancers rely on estrogen to induce breast cancer cell growth. Hormone therapy is provided to stop estrogen from binding to areas of the body where cancer cells can spread. Male hormone and androgen both contribute to cancer cell development. Limiting the levels of both estrogen and androgen is thus essential to reduce the spread of cancer cells.

A biological response modifier is used to activate the body's immune system for cancer control in biological therapy. It helps to improve the natural protection of the body against particular diseases such as cancer. Biological therapy remains in clinical trials, however.

You don't want to reach these stages of any kind of cancer. That is why it is extremely important that you go to a doctor as soon as possible if you see any of the above cancer signs manifesting. Listen to the body "speak" and follow the signs.

BREAST CANCER-A GROWING THREAT TO MEN AND WOMEN

Think of breast cancer and, of course, people think about a condition that is women's number one illness. But the truth is that breast cancer in women and men is growing, and experts find the national obesity crisis to be the blame.

We should probably expect more cancers linked to obesity with two-thirds of Americans now overweight. On the lighter side, though, weight problems can be handled well and even avoided. In the degree that overweight leads to cancer, this is one risk factor that we can actually control.

Nonetheless, how we gain that power seems important. Even among the most inspired, we see very few of people succeed in their individual attempts to lose weight, even if their lives depend on it. And it obviously does benefit cancer patients.

Take some of the figures: In women, breast cancer rose by 52 percent between 1973 and 1998. Much of this change can be explained by better detection, as mammography is much more available than 30 years ago. But it has also become common to use postmenopausal estrogen supplements that are specifically linked to cancer in women.

In the same time period, the prevalence of breast cancer in men increased by 26%, without the ingested estrogen and the additional mammography detection, since men do not usually follow this protocol.

So what else is happening? Experts believe the rise in breast cancer in both genders seems to follow closely the spike in US obesity, contributing to the hypothesis that the obesity crisis could be the cause of the breast cancer boom.

Obesity has shown a clear relationship to some, but not other, cancers. For example, there seems to be no link between men's overweight and prostate cancer. Or the relationship is sometimes obvious, but the motives aren't.

Researchers are therefore investigating whether acid reflux can account for the increased incidence of esophageal cancer in overweight people.

But there is at least one known reason for breast cancer: too much estrogen. In both men and women, fatty tissue contains estrogen.

Menopausal women's studies demonstrate the case most clearly. The ovaries are the primary source of hormones until menopause. But after menopause, once ovaries have withdrawn, the main source of estrogen is fatty tissue.

Estrogen levels among postmenopausal women are 50 to 100 percent higher in heavy women than those of healthy weight. Different ratios between men are noticed.

And when the tissues resistant to estrogen become more exposed to estrogen, this leads to the development of breast-responsive estrogen tumors.

Researchers estimate that the 11,000 to 18,000 deaths from breast cancer per year in American women aged over 50 years can be prevented if they maintain a healthy body weight during their adult lives. Men do not have the same statistics because, while breast cancer is a growing problem for men, there are few studies into male mortality rates and even less than cardiac disease or prostate or colon cancer.

Nevertheless, obesity often puts men at greater risk for these diseases, so the excess weight, or some of it, must be reduced. There is plenty of evidence that even a small weight loss has huge health benefits. How do you do that, then?

It is difficult, especially if you are older, and the average diagnosis age of 62 among women and 67 among men is for breast cancer.

Motivation is important, but research shows that it's not sufficient. People need assistance. For example, who would be more motivated to lose weight than a heavy person with cancer?

An overweight survivor has a double whammy for the possibility of recurrence, but a study published earlier in Obesity Research this year said that people left to their own devices or who only had a group plan did not achieve much weight loss even among that motivated group.

For those of us who have treated obesity for years, that is no surprise. We see people who tried to cook, went to the gym and the club and communion, all in vain. But if equipped with an intensive diet and lifestyle change plan that is specifically designed for them, things change.

In a recent study, researchers were quite unambiguous and concluded that 'for survivors of breast cancer to lose weight to reduce risk factors, intervention is needed. Of the various intervention regimes, individualized therapy combined with a weekly participation... was most successful....' Without a proper retraining, even the greasiest burger is difficult to match a lethal tumor. Nonetheless, professional support makes the difference.

For example, in weight management patients, I track levels of insulin for years since we know that high levels of insulin indicate a metabolic abnormality that leads to diabetes and weight gain. Recent research has now shown that high insulin levels are also a risk factor for recurrence of breast cancer.

Yet very specific changes in lifestyle and diet can reduce insulin levels dramatically in days or weeks, reducing the risk of the disease instantly. The risk of disembodied diseases is sometimes difficult for people to understand, but when clinicians can look at the results of their study and see how their behavior change affects their blood chemistry directly, it makes sense.

It happens to patients' bodies inside them. When they lose weight, it is more critical than improvements outside, but they will not have an opportunity to understand that even in the best health clubs and peer support groups.

It's exciting to see how people use a health and weight-loss system when they have more than just a bathroom scale to prove it works. Consistent and reliable guidance is crucial, since nobody goes from obese to safe overnight. Time is needed.

Yet cancer still takes time, so the race starts. With the right help, this is a competition that men and women are very likely to win.

The most common disease among women is breast cancer, and it is the second leading cause of death from cancer, which was surpassed by lung cancer only in 1985. Sometime in her life, one woman in eight who lives to the age of 85 develops breast cancer.

Currently, more than 2 million women in the US are treated for breast cancer. Approximately 41,000 people will die of the disease. The risk of breast cancer death is about 1 in 33. Nevertheless, the death rate from breast cancer is increasing. The decline was probably due to early detection and better therapy.

Breast cancer is not just an illness of a woman. The American Cancer Society reports that 1600 people develop the disease annually, and approximately 400 men will die.

The risk of breast cancer is greater among those who have breast cancer before the age of 50. If you have breast cancer only with a mother or sister, your risk doubles. For two first-grade relatives diagnosed, the risk increases to five times the average.

Although the cause of breast cancer is not known exactly, sometimes the culprit is an inheritable mutation in one of two genes, BRCA1 and BRCA2. Such genes usually protect against the disease by generating protein that prevents irregular cell growth, but the risk of breast cancer can rise by 80 per cent for women with the mutation, up to 13 per cent of the population. In reality, over 25% of women with breast cancer have a history of the disease in their families.

The threats are harder to identify in women without a family history of breast cancer. Hormone estrogen is known to feed some breast cancers; various factors –diet, excess weight and consumption of alcohol –may increase body estrogens.

Early signs: Early signs of breast cancer include: a lump that is usually single, solid and generally painless.

The skin layer on the breast or the underside of the leg is swollen and appears odd.

Veins become more pronounced on one breast on the skin surface.

The affected breast nipple is twisted, develops acne, changes the texture of the skin or has a release other than breast milk.

A depression develops on the surface of the breast.

Breast cancer forms and stages: There are many different types of breast cancer. Some are rapidly growing and volatile, while others mature faster and steadier. Some are stimulated by body estrogen; some are the result of mutation in one of the two genes mentioned above-BRCA1 and BRCA2.

In-situ Ductal carcinoma (DCIS): Generally divided into a comedy (Blackhead) in which there is an extrusion of dead and necrotic tumor cells, similar to blackheads and non-comedos, on the cut tumor surface. DCIS is early breast cancer that is contained within the ductal network. It is important to distinguish comedy and no comedy forms because comedocarcinoma typically behaves more aggressively on the spot and may display areas of micro invasion of adjacent tissue through the ductal wall.

Ductal infiltration: This is the most common type of breast cancer and accounts for 78 percent of all diseases. These lesions can occur in the field of mammography in two different forms: star-like or well circumscribed (rounded). In general, star lesions have a poorer prognosis.

Medullary carcinoma: 15% of breast cancers are malignant. In particular, these lesions are small and difficult to differentiate by mammography or sonography from fibro adenoma. With this type of brain cancer, estrogen and progesterone receptor prognosis measures are negative 90% of the time. Medullary carcinoma is typically more severe than other forms of breast cancer.

Infiltration Lobular: Comprising 15% of breast cancer, these lesions usually appear as slight thickening in the upper surface of the breast, which is difficult to diagnose with mammograms. Both breasts can be involved in lobular penetration (bilateral). These tumors microscopically have a linear range of cells and grow around ducts and lobules.

Tubular carcinoma: This is defined as orderly or distinguished breast carcinoma. Such lesions account for approximately 2% of breast cancers. We have a good prognosis with a survival rate of almost 95% after 10 years.

Mucinous carcinoma: Represents 1-2 percent of breast carcinoma and has a good outlook. These lesions are usually limited (circumcised).

Inflammatory breast cancer: This is a very aggressive type of breast cancer, which is typically shown by skin changes such as redness, skin thickening, and the prominence of hair follicles that are similar to orange peel. The diagnosis is made by a skin biopsy, which shows tumors about 50% of the time in the lymphatic and vascular channels.

Breast cancer stages: Ductal carcinoma is the most common type of breast cancer. It starts with the lining of the ducts. In the lobules, another form, called lobular carcinoma, occurs. When cancer is detected, it is difficult for a pathologist to determine what cancer it is-whether it has started in a duct (ductal) or in a lobula (globe) and if it has reached surrounding breast tissues.

Specific laboratory tissue studies are usually performed to learn more about cancer when cancer is detected. For example, receptor tests for hormones (estrogen and progesterone) can help determine whether hormones help cancer to grow. If test results indicate that hormones have an effect on cancer growth (a positive test result), the cancer can respond to hormonal treatment. This treatment extracts hormones from the cancer cells.

Sometimes, other tests are done to help predict if the cancer is going to advance. Sources of this are x-rays and other laboratory tests. Sometimes, a sample of breast tissue is tested for a gene known as the human receptor-2 (HER-2 gene) epidermal growth factor that is associated with a greater risk of breast cancer recurrence. Special bone, liver and lung examinations are carried out because breast cancer can spread to these areas.

The treatment options for a woman depend on a number of factors. These factors include age and menopausal status, general health, tumor size, location, cancer stage, laboratory test results, and breast size. Other characteristics of tumor cells are also considered, such as whether they rely on hormones to develop.

The most important factor in most cases is the phase of the disease. The stage depends on the tumor size and whether the cancer has spread. The following are concise explanations of breast cancer stages and the therapies most commonly used for each stage. Sometimes, other treatments may be sufficient.

Phase 0: Step 0 is sometimes referred to as non-invasive carcinoma or in situ carcinoma. Lobular in situ carcinoma (LCIS) refers to abnormal cells in the lobule lining. Such abnormal cells are rarely invasive cancer. These are, however, an indication of an increased risk of breast cancer development in both breasts. LCIS is a drug called tamoxifen, which reduces the risk of breast cancer. A person who is affected can choose not to receive treatment but to monitor the situation through regular inspections. And sometimes, surgery is used to remove both breasts to try to prevent the development of cancer. In most instances, it is not necessary to remove the subarm lymph nodes.

Ductal in situ carcinoma (DCIS) refers to abnormal cells in a duct's lining. Intraductal carcinoma is also known as DCIS. The abnormal cells have not spread over the conduit to invade the breast tissue. People with DCIS are nevertheless at increased risk of invasive breast cancer. Many patients with DCIS were exposed to breast-saving procedure or radiation therapy. Instead, they can choose a mastectomy for reconstructing the breast with or without breast reconstruction (plastic surgery). Normally, hidden lymph nodes are not covered. Women with DCIS might also discuss tamoxifen with their physician to reduce the risk of developing invasive breast cancer.

Stages I and II: Stages I and Stages II are early stages of breast cancer, where the cancer spreads across the lobe or canal and has reached surrounding tissues.

Phase I means the tumor is one inch in size, and the cancer cells do not spread beyond the breast.

Stage II means the tumor in the breast is less than one inch in size, and the cancer has spread to the lymph nodes below the arm.

The tumor is 1 to 2 inches (with or without lymph node distribution under the arm).

The tumor is 2 cm larger but has not spread to the lymph nodes below the arm.

Early stage breast cancer treatment options include breast-saving procedure followed by breast radiation therapy and mastectomy with or without breast reconstruction to replace the breast. These methods also treat early-stage breast cancer. (Mastectomy is also used for radiation.) The option of breast-sparing surgery or mastectomy depends primarily on the size and location of the tumor, breast shape, other characteristics of the cancer and how the person feels about breast preservation. Typically, lymph nodes under the arm are extracted with either strategy.

Chemotherapy and/or hormone treatment are indicated in Stage I and most often in Stage II breast cancer following primary surgery or surgery and radiation therapy. This extra treatment is known as adjuvant therapy. Systemic treatment, also called neoadjuvant therapy, reduces the

tumor before surgery. This is done to destroy any
remaining cancer cells to prevent cancer.

Phase III: Phase III is also known as advanced regional
cancer. At this point, the tumor in the breast may display
the following: more than 2 inches across and the cancer
has spread to the lymph nodes of the underarm.

The cancer in the underarm lymph nodes is severe.

The cancer spreads to lymph nodes in the region of the
breastbone.

The type of locally advanced breast cancer is inflammatory
breast cancer. In this kind of cancer, the breast appears
red and swollen (or inflamed) because the lymph vessels in
the breast are blocked by cancer cells.

Phase III patients with breast cancer normally have both
regional care for breast cancer removal or death and
preventive medication to prevent the disease from
spreading. Local treatment may be breast or underarm
surgery and/or radiation therapy. Systemic therapy can
include chemotherapy, hormonal therapy, or both.
Systemic therapy can be used to shrink the tumor or to

stop the condition from occurring in the breast or elsewhere before regional treatment.

Stadium IV: Phase IV is metastatic. The disease has spread to other parts of the body beyond the breast and under armed lymph nodes.

Phase IV therapies for breast cancer include chemotherapy and/or hormonal therapy, which kills and controls cancer cells. Patients may have breast cancer surgery or radiation therapy. Radiation can also be effective in other parts of the body to suppress tumors.

Recurrent Cancer: Recurrent cancer means, despite the initial diagnosis, the disease has returned. Even if a breast tumor seems to have been completely removed or killed, sometimes the disease returns when undetected cancer cells linger in the body following treatment.

Many recurrences occur in the first two or three years following treatment, but breast cancer can recur for many years.

Cancer that only occurs in the surgical region is called local recurrence. If the disease spreads to another part of the body, it is known as metastatic breast cancer. The patient can have one type of therapy or a combination of repeated cancer treatments.

HOW TO CALCULATE YOUR RISK FOR BREAST CANCER?

Mathematical models can be developed using known risk factors for breast cancer to help answer important questions. To scientists and clinicians, these mathematical models are useful tools: 1. Risk factors study-The Claus risk assessment method has been used to evaluate the sub-population of those with a dominant autosomal genetic allele that increased their risk from 10% to 92%. It resulted in the discovery of BRCA genes for breast, ovarian, and prostate cancer.

2. Eligibility for a medical trial—A Gail risk assessment framework has been developed to help researchers decide who can participate in NSAPB Breast Cancer Prevention trials to minimize the risk of breast cancer chemoprevention.

3. Guidelines for BRCA testing–BRCA screening is very expensive and practically useful when performed on everyone (because it is so rare for BRCA1 and BRCA2 to be homozygous). Mathematical models, including BRCAPRO, BOADICEA, and Tyrer-Cuzick models, help to determine which patients should be screened for BRCA. The test decision is usually taken if one of these models predicts a 10 percent or more risk that BRCA1, BRCA2 or both genes will mutate.

4. MRI testing for breast cancer–MRI screening for breast cancer is not a cost-effective screening test for the general public, but strong explanations exist for specific groups. MRI screening for women with a 20-25 percent or higher risk of breast cancer is generally recommended. The BRCAPRO and Tyrer-Cuzick models were used to help make medical decisions on the ordering of MRIs for the screening of breast cancer.

5. Breast cancer recommendations — The Gail model is used medically to assess who should be used to avoid tamoxifen and tamoxifen. Other models were used to help decide on the reduction of the risk of breast cancer with prophylactic mastectomy.

It is important to understand these models for these reasons. These models are referred to collectively as "risk evaluation tools." The following paragraphs summarize the most popular and widely used instruments of risk assessment. Note that none of these risk assessment methods is available to victims of breast cancer. No mathematical model of cancer risk assessment in cancer survivors was generally accepted.

The Gail model is a validated risk-assessment method that mainly focuses on non-inherited risk factors with limited information on family history. Experts from the National Cancer Institute and the National Surgical Adjuvant Breast and Bowel Project (NSABP) have developed this method to assist health providers to assess the risk of breast cancer and determine their eligibility for the breast cancer prevention study. This method helps to predict the risk of breast cancer for a woman over a five-year period and over the course of her life. It also contrasts the risk calculation of the woman with the average risk of a person of the same gender. The Gail Model is an online quiz with 13 interactive questions. This model is based on reported hazard statistics and methods from publications reviewed by experts and has been extensively tested for validity.

The main limit of the Gail model is the inclusion in paternal lines of only families of the first level, which results in a underestimated risk of 50% of cancer families, and disregards the age of breast cancer inception. In certain populations, such as obese patients, it can underestimate risk.

The NCI Risk Assessment Model is basically a condensed Gail model that also has race variables. Gender is a factor that determines the risk of breast cancer but is exempt from clinical trial eligibility. This tool is probably the most popular online, interactive threat calculator available to the public. The online quiz is a nine-point questionnaire with multiple factors that will provide a person with a potential five-year risk of sheep cancer and a lifetime risk of breast cancer.

The NCI framework does not take into account other risk factors that can be adjusted. This experiment is therefore difficult to use as a motivational tool to show people how lifestyle can alter their risk of breast cancer. This can also not be used in women with DCIS, LCIS, or those who bear one of the BRCA genes in breast cancer survivors.

BRCAPRO model: This is a computer-displayed statistical model using two different algorithms for analyzing family history and helping a physician assess the possibility of either having a BRCA1 mutation or a BRCA2 mutation in a population. The findings can be used to assess if BRCA tests were suggested. This is very helpful given the high cost of BRCA ($3,000) analysis. None of the non-inherited risk factors can be included in the model. The BRCAPRO model is the least accurate when comparing four different methods for predicting the risk of breast cancer in patients with a family history of breast cancer. This predicted only 49 percent of breast cancer in the screened group of patients with a family history of breast cancer.

Harvard Center for Cancer Risk Assessment Tool: This is an additional tool for evaluating breast cancer risk that incorporates more lifestyle factors than the NCI and Gail template models. It has not been researched as thoroughly as the Gail Model or the simpler NCI, but it is interesting because it involves several lifestyle factors to change people's cancer risk. It is also an anonymous survey that both women and men can use to predict their risk of breast cancer.

Now that all these mathematical models have been explored extensively, it is time to make this data practical. How can a woman accurately determine the risk of breast cancer and tell, if possible, what positive factors reduce the risk and what negative factors can be adjusted to reduce the risk? Wherever possible, the value and indications for testing, imaging, chemoprevention, and in some cases surgery could also be shown to the patient. A review of each of these practical aspects is given in a Q&A format:

Q: Which (free) online services can be used to help a person assess his or her risk of breast cancer?

A: Several of the abovementioned risk assessment methods can be used by the public for free. The measures and their pages are as follows: 1. Your disease risk: This is a broad interactive questionnaire measuring the five-year and lifetime breast cancer risk developed by the Harvard Cancer Prevention Center released online in 2000. In 2005, the Spanish edition of "Cuidar de su Salud" was released. The hazard calculator covers indicators of lifestyle, such as weight, diet, consumption of alcohol, and Jewish ethnicity. However, this does not include other ethnic groups and is not true for BRCA carriers or survivors of breast cancer. Despite these issues, this is the best free online risk calculator because the computer is interactive and gives you a personalized description of your risk as a colored bar graph. The bar charts are seven-level, contrasting users to a typical man or woman of your age. Using tailored approaches, consumers learn where they can concentrate their prevention efforts and how to make lifestyle changes. The bar graph shrinks with each click, and the consumer watches his expected hazard fall. This is a great concept for inspiring people to take part and to adopt lifestyle changes.

2. This is the easy to use online questionnaire based on an updated Gail template that also involves ethnicity. The NCI Risk Assessment Tool does not affect the personal history of breast, DCIS, or LCIS cancer. Other factors, like BRCA status, hormones, life-style factors, breastfeeding, menopause, or mammographic density, are not taken into account. Despite these problems, it is a useful tool that gives a woman her lifetime risk of breast cancer for five years. It is the only resource that can be used by mobile handheld devices (any type). You can also install a version of this for PDAs with the Windows Pocket PC operating system.

Q: What programs can help a doctor decide on a MRI breast order?

A: The American Cancer Society has provided some good guidance on MRI testing for breast cancer. It should be emphasized that MRI is an improvement to mammography, not a replacement. Many software can be used in the decision-making process. Please check the website of the American Cancer Society.

Husbands: 10 reasons to be with your wife with breast cancer. Once we marry the man or woman of our dreams, our partner and best friend, we hope to be together for a lifetime despite the odds of being divorced being 6 in 10 marriages. They truly think that, "until death they are part of it, for the wealthy, the poor, sickness and health," we will be together. And then life comes into being: becoming a family, learning to balance needs, joy and the enormous obligation to be parents, managing jobs and money.

If a relationship is safe, a storm will withstand almost any trauma. If the relationship is not strong, a trauma, almost any trauma or pressure, will cause it to disappear. This may be because nearly seven in ten marriages that are affected by breast cancer do not survive.

There is no magic bullet, no panacea or mechanism for it to survive and actually thrive despite or, in part, because of the diagnosis and treatment of breast cancer and subsequent life together.

It is said that we have struggles to create character, so that you as a husband and you as a couple have a great chance to build character and create a lifetime love story. Shirley, fought breast cancer for 22 years. That doesn't define her, however. She is also a mom, a businessman, a teacher, a wife, a volunteer in the community and my life partner. At age 37, she was treated for stage 3 resistant tumor with significant involvement in the lymph node. She is alive and well, still sexy with just one breast and inspires other women, especially young women, who face this illness.

Below are tips to other husbands on how to become a survivor for your wife, how to support her.

1. Tell her you love her.

Silence is not golden in a marriage or any intimate relationship. The strong silent guy doesn't apply to a woman with breast cancer, father, boyfriend, best friend, confidant, and supporter. Your daughter, your girlfriend, needs you and wants to hear you. Actions may talk more clearly than words, and you may do the right things, but words give comfort, reassurance, and awareness of your inner feelings. She cannot read your mind. It is more than physical and economic security to be there for her. Words have meaning. At the moment, when you together face her death, the three key words are: "I love you." The late, Louise Crisafi, who always gave herself on Earth to others in need, taught me this lesson on Friday, when my mother, Shirley Ann, was diagnosed with her biopsy. Every day, Shirley had chosen a two-step diagnostic process, and on the second day, Shirley decided to treat her right breast surgery, a mastectomy. That means we knew Friday that on Monday, after a weekend together, she would have a mastectomy. She was terrified, nervous and afraid. Shirley faced her death and the inevitable loss of her femininity. I felt confused, overwhelmed, and scared, at a loss. I didn't know what to do or say.

Louise was a fundraiser from the American Cancer Society to help other women face the diagnosis and treatment of breast cancer. She was a good friend. As I asked her what to do, she said simply: "Tell her that you love her." I was off at the races. That weekend, I said these three magic, powerful words over and over, perhaps more often than I had done in weeks, months and years.

A year or so ago, Shirley recalled how verbalized I became this fateful weekend, during a Television talk show featuring three women who had breast cancer. Those phrases are soothing and shifting. Remember to say, "I love you." And I hope that today I am as verbal and loving as I am in the middle of a crisis.

2. We all know the joke about Moses and the tribes of Israel that wandered through the desert for 40 years after their miraculous escape from the bondage of Egypt. The land of milk and honey, the Promised Land, took 40 long years. And why did it take so much time? Moses was a man. He refused to ask for help. Ten Commandments, perhaps, never asking for help.

If you've been married and dating a guy for a long time, you've lost time in a car. You say, maybe timidly and quietly, that stopping and asking for directions could be a good idea. He is insulted. He is offended. He's a kid, after all. He's got a good sense of direction. That's going to be clear to you, a dumb girl, without a sense of direction. The moments are over. He gets exasperated and hits the ignition. Finally, he pulls into a gas station and asks for help in disgust. It scares him to do that.

Louise added a further lesson when I asked what I could do, realizing that both Shirley and I were facing her cancer together. Her advice was insightful and powerful. If anyone asks if they can do anything to help, just say "yes."

Parents, family, neighbors, employers, etc. want to be there for themselves and for you.

I know, you are a person and never ask for help, not even basic advice. Understand that those who ask to help need your "Yes" as much as you do. It gives them a feeling that they can do something positive about this insidious disease that appears beyond their control.

Shirley and I have been fortunate. We did not have to cook a meal for three to four months after her surgery because of the chicken dishes, casseroles, lasagnas and other goodies that streamed continuously through our window. It was there for our friend, Alison, to need a brief childcare stint. Thanks, Greenwich. Thank you. Many gratitude to First Congregational Church in Old Greenwich in particular. Thank you very special friends, especially Betsy, who taught me that I could do anything, even that. You are a family of empathy. You're a priest of salvation. You are true friends. Your compassion, prayers and support have led to our healing for all three of us.

Please ask for help. If offered, say "yes." You will be better for it.

3. Humor Heals: Norman Cousins taught the country this lesson many years ago, and Loretta Laroche and others often remind us of this truth. We know that laughing is soothing. It gives us a better feeling and allows us to improve. We are very quick to get too critical of ourselves and our careers.

Close friends have witnessed our sporadic over - the-top laughter out of control. Can anything feel better? You can't laugh while you're sorry. Seeing the humor brings relief and release in any situation. Have you ever heard of the driver, who has a "speeding" ticket after his car's wheel? Tragedy, yes. With retrospect, being able to laugh at the accident brings empathy and relaxation.

Our favorite apocryphal joke is to hit a cow, secretly report the accident and collect a $500 card via e-mail. Shirley set the stage for our approach to her breast cancer treatment, which included humor and many things. Shirley met her surgeon's wife, Linda McWhorter, about two weeks before her diagnosis and operation. On the way to the operating room for her mastectomy, sitting on the hangar of a local community hospital, she looked up and said, "Hey, Phil, you ought to charge me half the price."

A year ago, Shirley told the President and CEO of the hospital that she was overcharged for her mammogram to have a 50% discount. After all, they had only to take one x-ray of one remaining breast, not two. What is fair being fair. It is equal. She left him voiceless. It was only important to me.

And her oncologist, Dick Hollister, and his outstanding team have been there. Did you know that over 95% of cancer treatment is in the private office of doctors, not in hospitals? When you choose to study oncology, at least 50 percent of your patients will die there. Nevertheless, Dick and his team always gave hope, warmth and, of course, fun and humor.

According to his wife, at age 11, Dick decided to become a doctor and treat patients with cancer at the age of 13. Shirley was the perfect match when she whispered her temporary prosthesis during her first visit to her hospital room, turning her bright red (fairly easy, because of her shocking red-hair). He was speechless. He realized that he had one life, despite the poor forecast. In his first few years of practice, Shirley was an interesting and challenging case for a young oncologist. During our year of therapy, jokes were a staple in his office.

Humor is body, mind and spirit healing.

4. Despite growing obesity, we are a body and breast image culture, from Betty Grable's World War II pinups to Marilyn Monroe and Jane Mansfield in the 1950's and 1960's to Salma Hayek, Paris Hilton, and Pamela Anderson today. I love you. Men talk about being bravely and sophomoric "leg men" or "breast men," as though large breasts and big legs have to do with being a woman, a lifetime partner, and a long-term lover.

Don't get me wrong. I love to look at and respect beautiful women from the glamorous 76-year-old model who brought my 1982 smoking-cessation to the stars on the television and women today around me. Nevertheless, my physical and sensual desire is my wife, my lover and my lifelong partner today. Your bride, your wife should know how much you care about them, not what kind of body they have or their breast size.

Shirley is as gorgeous and sexy today as she was, if not more, on our first date. Our passion wasn't and is not hampered by having one breast instead of two. It enriches our friendship instead. She completes me when we make love, makes me whole and alive. God created a set that fits nicely together. Your bride needs confidence in the face of an assault on her femininity. She needs to know by what you say and do that this set of circumstances is not the end of your sex life but a new sex life of greater sensitivity and care, which is sometimes frightful and thrilling.

5. Go to her appointments and hold her hand, literally and figuratively, with as many meetings as you can with your wife and mother. In my job as CEO of the health and wellness center, I had the luxury and blessing of relative independence. I have built my family and professional schedule around Shirley's course of care. I attended nearly every doctor, every chemotherapy consultation, with Shirley. I was a little embarrassed that I was alone in the waiting room, not going for the actual treatments to the examination room with her. Perhaps somewhat wimpy or squashy, but every step of the way, I was with her in heart, body and spirit. I'd have taken it for her if possible and have traded places with her.

It's not what you do when you accompany her for treatment, but the act itself that tells her volumes. This gives you a sense of pride as well. You are more than a mere spectator who hates the wretched disease. You joined the struggle. You and your wife, family and friends, your treatment team and all the support systems around you help control the wrestling of cancer.

Hearing a cancer diagnosis overwhelms the senses. Doctors try to help you understand, but their everyday vocabulary, the medical language, can also be classical Greek or Latin. There are two sets of ears with you to hear what is said. Two eyes are open to ask questions. This helps to avoid the tendency to listen. Being with her will reassure her every time, help her to get over her fear, and make you feel good for yourself. She's going to love you for that.

6. Your wife or partner is not fragile. She's not an invalid. She's not going to break. Therapy can be tiring, but both of you need to live your life as fully as possible. Go on to enjoy what you enjoy individually and as a couple, especially as a couple. One of our best friends and an inspiration to many came to their chemotherapy meetings when they were fighting breast cancer recurrence. It is called zest to live; it's in the present.

Let your bride do whatever she can. In the case of Shirley during her year of treatment, this included hiking at Greenwich Point, skiing, playing golf with me, putting flowers and even sometimes agreeing to sail with me. You should take your questions from her. She knows what she can do or how exhausted she can be, whether or not it's a good day. If she's prepared, support her without pressuring her. Get out when she is ready.

As I see it, it was necessary that Shirley and I live completely with Alison as a couple and as a family. We realized that our time here together could be very short and that we wanted to live our lives completely together. We didn't anticipate the span of our life with which we were blessed. Shirley is a blessing, and so is your spouse or girlfriend, regardless of the ultimate result.

7. Sex After Breast Cancer: This is another area where a person must be allowed to lead his wife. They will let you know what's going on, what she's up for and what she's not. I guess I mourned her breast loss as she mourned the change in some facets of love-making.

The main thing to learn is that life continues and sex continues. Your sex life can take on an added dimension in the first weeks, months and even years, which is both frustrating and sublime. Imagine how you feel loving someone you might lose. You don't want to hurt her. You don't. She's not weak, remember. You can hug her during and outside your lovemaking.

Shirley found a new gynecologist, Ed Jacobson, a man whose presence and disposition were obviously soothing and restorative. It has enriched our lives by proposing that we seek jellies and creams to make our relationship easier and more relaxed. If the wife has menopause, whether as she ages spontaneously or, as in the case of Shirley, early menopause at the age of 37 with chemotherapy or hormone therapy, problems have to be addressed. It includes hot flashes, vaginal dryness, sexual discomfort, lack of lubrication, diminished libido. In describing Shirley's use of jellies and creams during an office visit, Ed described it as "the stuff used by prostitutes in Stamford." And it works, by the way.

Sex after mastectomy is beautiful, and it can be sublime and painful at the end. There is nothing that can prepare a person to love and to have a relationship with the love of his life, which he believes is lost. The danger that stood over our heads and for days, months and years were part of our thinking. Shirley would be ashamed if I said anything more about our sex life. It's personal and a treat.

I spoke to women's groups and social workers on this issue. The most rewarding thing was that I was in a panel in Stamford, Connecticut with a sex therapist talking to me. I listened carefully and was happy to find that Shirley and I worked out what she technically described on our own. She was a theoretician who explained the concepts of sexuality and the implications of breast surgery and cancer treatment. Shirley and I had experienced it and were just fine, thank you.

8. You need to understand that your husband, your wife, the wife you promised to cherish, the love of your life and your best friend are also the answers for your mid-life caricature. The response is not a young intern with a thong young enough to be your wife. It's not a young bimbo or colleague who starts your next marriage or family. This isn't a sports car, a speedboat, or a new golf club. It is your girlfriend. It's your mother.

After more than four decades of marriage, I met this attitude and understanding, observing the marriage of friends Joe and Shirley, two "adolescents in charity." Rather than have an alternative relationship with your girlfriend, whether sexual or emotional, take her to a cozy bed and breakfast for a relaxing weekend. In our situation, it could be a quiet time to paddle a canoe together in Berkshires. And take a Broadway show or a good film and a dessert after the show. Fall in love. Stay in love. Be in lust.

9. Lemonade from lemons: Make lemonade if life gives you lemons. See the silver lining. You are not a Pollyanna to seek something beautiful, dark and meaningful in the face of illness, death and loss. Would you see yourself in a cancer person's shoes or psyche? Or as a woman with breast cancer's husband, lover, and life partner? Do you deeply understand how intimate you are, whether physical or otherwise, as all your senses are stretched and stimulated by the awareness that you give love to a woman you might lose?

You find happiness to the point of pain. You experience a deep sense of being with each other, and you know that it can be transitory and passing. The truth can break in and break the moment, but you continue. Over the years, after "our" diagnosis for Shirley's breast cancer, I have often said that a strong matrimony or a solid bond is not just going to get through the ordeal of breast cancer. Your marriage is going to be improved and stronger. Go figure.

10. A man attending a support group for prostate cancer expressed concern that "damaged goods" would arise during prostate cancer treatment. With or without breast reconstruction, your bride is not harmed. She remains the one you have fallen in love with, the one you have been committed to together for life. Get beyond your inner thoughts, wondering if your lovemaking was forever changed. You too may miss her breast, because in the past it gave both of you pleasure. Whether or not breast reconstruction is a personal choice, your choice. Shirley decided not to do so, partly to avoid further disruption and "wakening" of missing cancer cells.

3 WAYS TO REDUCE BREAST CANCER RISK

Breast cancer has been associated with three factors: 1. Natural (body-produced) and synthetic (environmental chemicals) exposure to estrogen (hormone).

2. The way the liver breaks down and treats them.

3. The pace at which these substances are extracted from the intestine.

Across three ways, they can minimize or reduce the risk of developing breast cancer:

1. Minimizing artificial estrogen exposure.

2. Hold our liver clean and function well.

3. Keep our bowels and colon (good) healthy and working well.

How can we do that? Okay, synthetic estrogen is present in plastically packaged foods; in unfiltered tap water, household cleaners and meal, among other items, in soft plastic containers such as food storage containers, cling films, plastic shelves, etc. Synthetic estrogen can affect the breast tissue up to 100 times more than natural estrogen. We can support ourselves and our friends by trying to cut the plastic wrapping, buy a cart or a shopping bag or buy food from local produce shops or fishmongers / markets, ask the food to be put in your cart or a box or shopping bag directly. You must note that half of the dustbin is packed with plastic bottles, dots and wrappings. By cutting these plastics, you can simultaneously help the environment. When you are making your lunch for work and lunch for children, prepare food with grease-proof paper and paper bags. You can also save small glass containers for your luncheon. (Glass baby bottles are now available if you're thinking about that). Exposure to synthetic estrogen can also be limited by a water filter that uses eco-friendlier cleaning products, consumes less red meat, and prefers organic foods-especially organic food that contain less hormones and chemicals-that also uses less plastic to cover. The harmful effects of estrogen are also claimed to be offset by eating some soy products, which can add soy milk, soy yogurts and puddings, tofu sauces, soybeans and soybeans to your diet.

The second way to reduce our risk of breast cancer is to help our liver break down the estrogen in our body. In order to do so, you must reduce the amount of alcohol. The government recommendation on the healthy alcohol limit is 14 units for a woman every week and 21 units for men, but we suggest that our intake be lowered to several units a week by the association for awareness of breast cancer. Reducing your intake of alcohol will keep you happier for longer. Many medications used to help breast cancer livers are made from broccoli, and cruciferous vegetables (broccoli, chocolate, cauliflower and sprouts) can prevent cancer. It improves liver health by eating lots of fresh steamed broccoli. We are also able to promote liver health by consuming sufficient water, increasing our salt intake, avoiding cured or smoked food and meat, and regularly exercising and preventing recreational drugs and excessive medication. The liver can also be put under pressure by contaminants, such as paint fumes, aerosols and home chemical products, so masks are used in decorating and children are shielded from smoke. Avoid the use of chemicals when cleaning and pick more gentle items like Ecover. Use traditional methods such as soda bicarbonate and vinegar to wash glass-ask your mother and grandmother for hot tips!

The third way you can restrict your risk factors is to promote intestinal or intestinal health and quickly move unhealthy substances from the body (stay regular). We can do it in various ways- eat high-fiber foods, plenty of complex carbohydrates, lots of fruit and vegetables including meat, drink plenty of water, and exercise. All these components should stop the waste products in the intestine from flowing around the body and get them out faster, reducing the chances of estrogen breakdown that causes body damage. Maintaining our gut safety requires maintaining a healthy intestinal flora (friendly bacteria). This can be done largely with a diet rich in fruits and vegetables, milk, organic dairy, and alcohol avoidance.

Some of you reading this will already have breast cancer, and many improvements in diet and exercise can boost healing and reduce the likelihood of cancer. Recent studies have found that women who have already done multiple hours of workouts a week are likely to recover better from breast cancer, and women who have been doing moderate workouts for half an hour three days a week are more likely to recover more quickly and survive breast cancer. The consumption of complex carbohydrates, lots of fruit and vegetables and soybeans, will also help to recover, with balanced diets helping to cope with the fatigue of treatment. Smooth exercise helps to reduce the stress associated with cancer, and people suffering from it can benefit from relaxation, yoga, meditation, Tai Chis and prayer to alleviate stress and tension. Those with or wanting to avoid breast cancer will benefit from a strong anti-oxidant diet, such as broccoli, red, yellow and orange peppers, apricot, beetroot, spinach and chard, mango and papaya, cherries and carottes, blueberries and strawberries. Brazil Nuts is another super food that contains a potent anti-oxidant called selenium. Healthy eating and adaptive levels of activity performed on cancer treatments will help the body recovery and chemotherapy and surgery rehabilitation. Call the Bristol Cancer Help Center, a popular world organization that helps people recover, for more information and support on food.

Finally, here are some ways to help your body (and the bodies of those you care for) prevent and heal from breast cancer.

Regular self-monitoring and breast checks, notifying physicians of any abnormal changes.

Cut down on plastic bags, plastic bags and chemicals for washing.

Eat less meat and pick organic meat. Swap meat for a good protein source for soy products and offset the harmful effects of artificial food.

Cut down the intake of alcohol.

Eat complex carbohydrates and many fresh and colorful fruits and vegetables.

Take regular exercise-for those suffering from breast cancer 3x 30 minutes and, for all others, 3-4 hours a week.

The workout must not be boring and may be divided into small useful bits, a 20-minute walk to the park and 10 minutes of gardening, happily vacuuming with loud music for 15 minutes!

 Keep a healthy weight.

Remove pressure from your life as much as possible. Try to organize yourself as this can help. Find time to take care of yourself and relax. Try yoga, meditation and tai chi–many lessons, books and videos are available. Get stress out through gentle exercises, a candle-lighted tub, or watch a crying or funny film-anything that works for you. Remember that your body and mind should be comfortable and healthy.

Breastfeeding your babies reduces the risk for breast cancer.

If you can live in this manner, the risk of contracting many other tumors and other chronic conditions, including heart disease, will be minimized as much as possible. Providing children and grandchildren with a good example of healthy living can reduce their risk of suffering from chronic diseases later.

External radiation treatment System, Example of a prostate cancer ultrasound (ultrasound can be used for guidance for a biopsy): For example, a gland in the male reproductive system produces cancer through the tissues of the prostate, as cells mutate and spread uncontrollably.

These can spread to other parts of the body (especially the bones and lymph nodes) by migrating from the prostate.

Prostate cancer develops regardless of benign prostatic hypertrophy (or adenoma of the prostate). It is adenocarcinoma in the vast majority of cases.

Prostate cancer can lead to pain, urinary difficulty, erectile dysfunction, and other symptoms. Replacement is done by surgery, radiation therapy, hormone treatment, and sometimes chemotherapy.

Frequency: Breast cancer rates vary widely worldwide. It is less common in South Asia and Far East, more common in Europe and in the US. Breast cancer is rare among Asians and more common among Blacks, according to the American Cancer Society (high rates may also be affected by increased detection effort).

Prostate cancer most often occurs in people over 50 years. This is the most common type of cancer in men, where it kills more than any other cancer (except lung cancer). However, most people who develop symptoms of prostate cancer do not undergo treatment and die for other causes. Some genetic factors, toxicological factors and dietary factors seem to be involved in the development of the cancer.

We find out that cancer cell outbreaks occur between 30 and 70 percent in studies of men 70 to 80 years; prostate cancer is the most asymptomatic. The likelihood of a man 50 years old who is diagnosed with prostate cancer is just 10 percent. This cancer is lethal in 3% of cases.

Prostate cancer geography: The definition of this cancer varies greatly, which seems to be more prevalent in black people or where the family is pathologically affected by this disease. While in Caribbean Cities, there were generally higher deaths due to cancer between 1983 and 2002, deaths due to prostate and stomach were twice as common in the Caribbean (although colorectal and lung cancer are three times less common). This may be explained by both genetic and dietary factors (green tea and/or soya or other selenium-rich foods), which seem to protect the majority of Japanese people living in Japan (while not resident in the US).

Causes: They are not properly identified.

The existence of certain genes seems to have a strong association with the development of the disease. In general, the higher incidence of this cancer in Black America could be explained by a mutation in chromosome 8.

A potentially protective function of lycopene has been explored with nutritional reasons. Likewise, exercise can have a slightly protective effect and smoking can cause damage.

Symptomatology and diagnosis: Prostate cancer is in most cases asymptomatic, i.e., it is detected if it does not have an occurrence of its own. It is most commonly found in blood tests, including PSA investigations (specific prostate antigen, whose predictive quality and use have recently been called into question without a proven benefit to public health). PSA is a protein that is normally isolated by prostate cells, but cancer cells are 10 times more secretive than normal cells. This estate has demonstrated several screening hopes. Blood PSA can be increased by many other factors (prostate size, infection and/or inflammation, mechanical (digital rectal other)) or reduced by some benign treatments (managed). Therefore, the levels of significance are difficult to determine. Nevertheless, PSA levels between 4 and 10 ng / ml are doubtful, but it is important beyond this. Several researchers recommended that the rate be taken to its true Prostate Weight or that the free PSA / total PSA or kinetic growth rate be measured over 2 years. Nevertheless, the PSA rate is still unclear for testing, and a key predictor of cancer detection and treatment is stated.

During a rectal examination on sections of prostate resection of prostate adenoma, which is performed as routine or due to other disease-related symptoms (especially benign prostatic hypertrophy).

The most advanced level is when symptomatic prostate cancer is detected. The clinical orientation is based on two key elements: the electronic rectal test and PSA blood determination: acute urinary retention, hematuria, sexual impotence, weakened general diseases, pain and/or malfunction or failure on the part of other organs linked to the presence of metastases. One or both of these anomalies causes suspected prostate cancer. It will be checked or not by taking a prostate specimen (biopsy) for microscopic examination. Only the optimistic nature of these biopsies helps this cancer to be detected and treated. We conduct a bone scan for bone metastases and abdominal-pelvic CT and MRI abdomino-pelvic once the diagnosis of prostate cancers is verified to clear tumor enlargement in prostate and in houses for potential pelvic metastases of the pelvic lymph node, retroperitoneal or liver.

Clinique: The basic digital rectal examination is the medical examination.

The most general induration of the gland can be nodular; it can include a whole lobe or the whole gland.
Heterogeneity or asymmetry are far less precise signs that

can also translate a simple adenoma, particularly when the prostate is bigger.

Ultrasound trans-rectal biopsies: No imaging procedure is available that can only detect a prostate adenocarcinoma outbreak with sufficient sensitivity and specificity.

In contrast to the common belief, this examination and endorectal ultrasound still commonly recommended alone is not important for the positive diagnosis of prostate cancer but is likely to cause disadvantages. This shall, however, be used to direct prostate biopsies when it's used. Other imaging techniques (scan, MRI) have an interest in the expansion of the balance sheet.

Technique: An endorectal ultrasound probe is inserted into the rectum with a guide needle. Biopsies with needles fitted with a leaned mandrel are carried out. The first one penetrates the mandrel. The needle literally covers and arrests the prostate break in the spot. A series of springs automates the motion of the chuck and the needle and takes several hundredths of a second. The ultrasound monitor, with a symbol indicating the direction of the needle, allows for very accurate biopsy.

The number and location of biopsies are not fully codified, and many protocols have been proposed; the objective is to obtain a sample that is as representative as possible. Usually, 5 to 6 specimens are per lobe and 10 to 12 in total, depending on the size of the penis, or the patient's sensitivity, or if a second set of biopsies.

Preparedness and quality: This is often achieved as an ambulator, i.e., without hospitalization, or during "day" hospitalization. A rectal preparation (enemas) is often recommended. Several centers are now providing systemic antibiotics (short treatment of antibiotics to eliminate infectious complications). By practice, concomitant anticoagulation is ineffective, and any treatment may be subject to arrest or immediate alteration.

The approval of the test is especially variable from patient to patient. Each biopsy is very painful. Their repetition, in particular the presence and movement of the sensor, is the main reason for discomfort. The drawbacks of this review may justify the use of local or general anesthesia. Local gel anesthesia (lidocaine gel) has never shown efficacy. Local lidocaine injection (pudendal nervosity) on both sides of the prostate demonstrated increased sensitivity of the exam in many trials, although incomplete due to its low-efficiency pain, related to the presence of the specimen. The recently tested mild equimolar oxygen and nitrous oxide mixture ("MEOPA") tends to be very active in this instance. It's even more fascinating, because it doesn't need an anesthetist and seems almost without side effects. General "classical" anesthesia is commonly used in patients who have experienced significant pain during the first of a series of prostate biopsies.

Suites: The suffering will reduce in time. Little bleeding from anus and urine can occur fairly frequently for 24 to 72 hours without gravity. Small blood nets can also mess with semen for several days, with no consequences.

Anatomopathology: Cancer begins in the peripheral portion of the gland, as opposed to benign prostatic hypertrophy of central interest, periuretral.

The diagnosis relies on the biopsy or surgical sample analysis.

The gravity of evolution is linked to the microscopic appearance (Gleason score), the PSA level, and disease spread.

Extension of the balance: The propagation of infection allows for personalized treatment, when the illness has to be decided. The involvement of bone metastases, lung, and liver is therefore the most common knowledge of bone metastases. Lymph node metastases in the pelvic and retrograde (round the abdominal aorta) must be examined. Finally, the extension of the tumor to the prostate must be clarified, in particular whether it exceeds the prostate capsule.

The imaging techniques used in routine usually show low capacity (ultrasound scan, MRI) and specifically identify the initial prostate lesions due to low blood levels of breast cancer. MRI is the least bad measure for the regional extension to be decided.

In order to achieve lymph nodes, MRI scanners and new generation (volume) are used, but only nodes whose size is increased are detected. The so-called "super-para-magnetic" products can boost the identification of damaged lymph nodes.

Yet, positron emission tomography (PET screen, PET scan) did not indicate very little or no prostate cancer due to hypermetabolism.

A blood test can check the status of the functions of the kidney and the liver.

Treatment Age, overall human health and the rate of spread, presence under the microscope, and cancer response to initial therapy are critical in predicting disease outcomes.

Because prostate cancer is an elderly male disease, many will die before prostate cancer can spread or cause symptoms for other reasons. This makes the choice of treatment complicated. To decide when we treat localized prostate cancer (a tumor that is located in the prostate) for therapeutic purposes, the positive and negative should be arbitrated from a point of view of patient safety and quality of life.

After the progression of cancer, the patient's general health and related illnesses, the diagnosis should be addressed case by case. A simple monitoring of the elderly or holders of a very localized person may be recommended.

Medical therapy hormone: There is a correlation between testosterone production (male hormone) and cancer cell multiplication. The disorder can be easily curbed if the hormone is blocked or greatly reduced. Many medications are given every 3 months as a subcutaneous injection. Others are orally handled. Nevertheless, the side effects are frequent but seldom severe. The hormone used to treat advanced forms or metastatic was applied to the treatment of tumors that were rejected for surgery (due to the tumor's volume, the likelihood of surgery was not complete,...), as well as the fact that relapse was essential after radiotherapy. Total disease control, with radiation therapy and hormone therapy applied every three years, could dramatically increase the number of patients whose illness remains undetectable. Since the 90s, pulpectomy (testicular ablation of tissue) has not been used.

Chemotherapy: Until the early 2000s, cytotoxic chemotherapy was not successful in metastatic prostate cancer and its common hormone treatment (especially increased PSA in spite of repeated androgen suppression). The introduction of docetaxel (Taxotere) changed the therapeutic possibilities, which was discovered some years earlier by mitoxantrone (Novantrone). A drug used for the first time in early stages of the disease has been able to improve patients ' longevity and quality of life. Such findings were confirmed by three controlled studies. Others are under way to integrate chemotherapy into the disease history of locally advanced tumors, where organic growth but before metastasis occurs, immediately after surgery to treat potential micrometastases.

Surgery: It is based on radical and complete prostatectomy. It involves removing the prostate and seminal vesicles and may be preceded by lymphatic prostate drainage levy. Operation can be done by means of opening (surgical incision in the abdomen or perineum) or abdominal coelioscopy; the surgery is reserved for cancer of the prostate and offers a large opportunity for cure if cancer is located and somewhat or moderately aggressive (Gleason score estimates aggressiveness) and can lead to urinary incontinence, usually temporary or erectile. There is currently no superiority of one technique over another in terms of cancer results and urinary and sexual function results.

Coelioscopy: Coelioscopy prostatectomy was used by an American team, which released it in 1997, after 8 cases, as it was difficult to intervene. The French teams took the torch at the end of 1997 and the beginning of 1998, showing that this technique was possible. Gaston de Bordeaux and VALLANCIEN Paris, and the technical standardization was established. VALLANCIEN and his group published the technique then through peritoneal, which looks simpler through transpéritonéale. It is now internationally remembered. The Montsouris Institute Surgical Group in Paris has undergone nearly 3 000 transactions and has shown the advantages of prostatectomy. Coelioscopy should maintain a shorter hospital stay (5 days vs 8 on average according to the PMSI 2004 statistics), a postoperative discomfort almost null, a transfusion rate of around 2 to 3 percent compared with average of 15 percent for open surgery. After about a week, activity resumption is rapid.

Cryoablation: A local application of a very cold gas may kill prostate cancer tissue. The cryoprobe (most commonly cooled with liquid nitrogen) is placed endourétrally on the prostate, and various procedures, such as endoscopy by a pubic trocard additive, are used to confirm the right cryode location. A freezing and thawing process will be applied for a few minutes, and a specimen is put uretrovésicale end technology if needed and enables progressive tissue necrosis to be evacuated by applying the cold, some training, cryotherapy-mortified tissue resection. Another strategy is to use a perineal ultrasound to put different needles under command.

The chances are very high that you or someone you meet has or will die of cancer. Following heart disease, cancer is the second most common cause of death in the United States. Males have significantly less than 1 in 2 lifetime cancer risk, whereas for women, the risk is slightly greater than 1 in 3.

All cancers involve gene malfunction to control cell growth and division. That cell in the body has a script, called the DNA or genetic code, that tells it what to do.

Mutations occur if the cell DNA code is modified a little by hormonal imbalances, chemicals, or free radicals. Cells with altered DNA don't look like the initial cells from which we were born. Mutations also increase with age, and about 78 percent of all cancers in people aged 55 and older were diagnosed.

Around 5% of all cancers are strongly inherited. Nevertheless, most cancers are not the product of inherited genes, but of DNA damage during one's lifetime.

We all have in our bodies a few cancer cells that are normally killed by our immune system. To hit the lump or bump level, it takes about a billion cancer cells, which means it takes years for a tumor to develop.

Cancer is a man-made illness in particular. You can do a lot now to reduce this risk dramatically. Know how many causes this disease can be associated with and how many dietary measures can reduce your risk of cancer.

Causing Factors: 1. Constant Emotional Pressure. The most important element of infection development is negative emotions. Even the CDC (Center for Disease and Prevention) states that 85% of the disease is psychological. If you are constantly angry, frightening, worried, cynical, discouraged or pessimistic, the body can create free radicals that cause DNA damage.

Look at your life closely and find anything out of order. If you have trouble dealing with it and resolving it yourself, look for professional assistance (such as a life coach or a therapist).

Do you always look at a half-empty glass? Changing your behavior from negative to positive can influence the situation and emotional results.

Learn to respect your emotions and be true to yourself rather than hide them by saying things like "I'm just fine." People who are able to express their feelings reduce stress in the body and are happier in general.

With a support system and safe pressure sources (such as exercising or playing musical instruments), mental wellbeing will always be so important.

With purpose, passion and gratitude, live your lives.

2. In today's world, we are constantly exposed to various environmental and food pollutants. Pollutants cumulate in the body. When these toxins enter the body, they build up (especially in fat cells) and produce huge amounts of free radicals that destroy the DNA in time. It is therefore important to identify them first and foremost and to prevent them.

Use of tobacco products and secondary smoke exposure, excessive sun exposure, household cleansers, air fresheners, bug sprays, soaps, personal hygiene products and cosmetics, excessive sun exposure, toxic chemicals.

Diagnostic tests such as CT scans, X-rays and mammograms create exposure to radiation. Try to minimize these tests and opt for MRI if you can afford it. Thermography, which identifies precancerous or cancerous tissues that are cold as opposed to hot benign lesions, is a much cheaper and more effective option. Sadly, not all insurance policies cover it.

Cell phone and cable phone electromagnetic radiation. Two recent long-term studies have found that cell phone radiation substantially increases the risk of gland salivary and brain tumors. For this reason, the use of the microphone, wired headsets and Bluetooth headsets (less radiation than mobile phones) is most effective. Seek not to explicitly keep mobile telephones to your ear.

Dietary toxins: In conventionally grown meat and farmed fish, pesticides and herbicides contain antibiotics and hormones. Where appropriate, select natural, herbal meats (organic meats are the second best) or wild fish from clean, cold water. Fish caught in safe waters have no mercury, which is a brain toxin.

GMOs, such as canola oil and soy product, contracting agents and food additives, dried nitrate and nitrites in dried or smoked meats, MSG, oxidized and rancid fat in polyunsaturated soy, cotton, corn, sunflower and safflower oils. Such oils are rich in omega-6 fats and promote body inflammation. They are frequently found in processed food, fast food and food in the restaurant.

Charred and burnt foods carcinogens. Stop frying or baking. Boil, poach, boil, or roast at or below 300 degrees F, instead.

Artificial sweetening agents, toxic gases from Teflon and other non-stick cookware, plastic water bottles of harmful chemicals that purge and contaminate the water. When you leave and refill the bottle in a hot car, the exposure is increased.

3. Extra pounds: It is vital to keep your weight stable during life. Two-thirds of Americans are overweight. Extra pounds increase the risk of various cancers, including breast, colon, esophagus, liver, pancreas and uterine diseases. Call me for a free telephone consultation on the Metabolic Typing Nutrition Program for help and support in healthy weight loss.

4. Hormonal imbalance: All of us have carcinogenic genes in our brains; they are like light switches. Unfortunately, these switches are turned off when we age as our hormonal production decreases. Of course, we put more stress on our hormonal system by not managing stress, eating badly, and consuming and living with chemicals.

In order to restore these cancer-protective genes, we have to live and eat better and restore the right balance of hormones. It is important that, when you substitute your hormones, you use a bio-identical hormone that is exactly the same as the hormones generated by your body and not the artificial hormones created by drug companies that cause cancer. You should consult a health professional with bioidentical hormone substitution therapy (BHRT).

Many hormones that have a direct effect on cancer growth are shown below: DHEA is a key hormone that reduces the amount of an important enzyme involved in the way that energizes cells in cancer. This route becomes less effective by keeping DHEA at the right level. Individuals who are under pressure continuously and who have fatigued adrenals have lower DHEA, which means they are more likely to promote cancer cell development.

Estriol is a soft estrogen by itself. But it is anti-carcinogenic and carcinogenic in the presence of other estrogens, such as estradiol and estrone. When we age, the body produces less estriol and can reduce the risk of cancer by adding proper amounts.

The correct balance between 2-hydroxyestrogen and 16 alpha-hydroxyestrogen is necessary, both of which are estrogen metabolites (the byproducts of estrogen in the urine). If there are more than two than sixteen, the risk of breast cancer is smaller. If the difference is more than 16 than 2, the risk is higher. This 2/16 ratio is the biggest factor in the risk of estrogen-sensitive cancer and can be totally modified by dietary procedures (see below).

2-methoxyestradiol is a very effective anti-cancer hormone produced by the body. The growth of fibroid cells in the uterus is also inhibited.

5. Excessive alcohol consumption: Evidence shows that women who consume more than 2 drinks a day significantly increase their levels of free iron (iron not protein-bound) in breast tissue. Free iron causes intense inflammation and free generation of radicals.

The consumption of iron does not, however, lead to the risk of breast cancer. It is a high intake of alcohol and excess estrogen that contributes to an increased incidence of invasive breast cancer.

6. Too much or too little exercise is important as it increases the supply of oxygen to cells. Normal healthy cells need enough oxygen to function properly, but only in anaerobic (no oxygen) environment can cancer cells multiply and prosper. Therefore, when you sweat, many toxins accumulated in the body are carried away, particularly the toxins in the fat cells.

That said, too much exercise is not helpful either because the body is constantly stressed, causing a huge amount of free radicals, which can lead to damage to DNA.

Diet that reduces cancer risk: Sugar consumption is limited as cancer cells ferment sugar to produce energy for growth and propagation. Sugar also generates excess insulin, which acts as a second stimulus to cell growth, cell division, and eventually cancer cell propagation. So, be careful how much sugar and refined carbohydrate (which behaves like sugar) you take at once as increased blood glucose means more insulin in your body.

Vitamin D3, the most active vitamin to prevent new cancers and suppress existing cancers by strengthening and improving the immune system, is the sun and/or supplements. When you raise your D3, ensure that your body has enough vitamin K as a group. K is a good source of green leafy vegetables, such as kale, spinach and collard greens, swiss chard, turnip greens, mustard greens and broccoli brussels.

Brassica vegetables increase the 2-hydroxyestrogen body level to reduce the risk of breast cancer. Eat 3 or more servings a week of broccoli, cauliflower, brussels sprouts, chocolate, collard greens, kohlrabi, rutabaga, turnips, bok choy, and mustard greens. You can also get the advantages of this indole-3-carbinol supplement.

A balance affects the level of cell growth by hormones called prostaglandins. More omega-3 fats and less omega-6 fats. Omega-3 fats reduce inflammation, while omega-6 fats increase inflammation. Fish caught in clean, cold waters and grass-fed meats are good sources for the 3s. Sadly, most cattle in the U.S. eat corn, and their meat and milk products are far lower in omega-6 fats.

Eat a wide variety of fruit and vegetables to get a healthy dose of different defensive antioxidants against free radicals. Do not rely on only one particular antioxidant.

Natural folic acid from green leafy vegetables are far superior to the artificial folic acid in fortified refined meal products to improve the body's natural defenses against cancer. Therefore, make sure you have enough vitamin B12 as folate works to protect DNA from damage. For plant foods, vitamin B12 is not present in the liver, beef, poultry, shellfish, fish, or dairy products, only in animal products.

Drink sufficiently fresh, filtered water every day, keeping the lymphatic system clear and detoxifying the skin. Drink 8 to 10 eight-ounce glasses a day for an average person.

Provide adequate protein all day long at every meal and snack to help the liver absorb contaminants from the bile. Protein also helps keep blood sugar levels even.

Raise the intake of fibers (soluble and insoluble) to lower the risk of colon, breast and prostate cancer. The goal is 40-50 grams per day, more than twice what the average American eats every day.

Finally, there was also compelling evidence for resveratrol an anticancer (in red wine but only in moderation), turmeric (in curcumin), green tea, grape seed extract, extract of granite, squirrel (in ointments, apples and raisins), combined linoleic acid (in grass-fed meats and its milk), lute Olin (in celery, green pepper, carrots, olive oil, thyme, rosemary and ginger).

To reduce your risk of cancer, avoid constant emotional stress, accumulation of toxins (environmental and dietary), extra pounds, hormonal imbalance, excessive alcohol consumption, and excessive or too little exercise.

Do: limit your intake of sugar, make sure you have enough vitamin D3, eat more Brassica, have greater omega-3 fats and less omega-6 fats, a large range of fruit and vegetables, have enough clean, water filtered, and protein and fiber.

Breast cancer is an increasing risk for both men and women and a disease that has a strong correlation with obesity. Fat produces excess estrogen; excess estrogen generates breast cancer. And on the other hand, weight loss reduces the risk of cancer. The data is clear, but it does not encourage the mission. Professional support- and the sooner the better- makes it easier and more effective.

www.ingramcontent.com/pod-product-compliance
Lightning Source LLC
Chambersburg PA
CBHW061727250726
48657CB00002B/811